BODY COACHING

30 DAYS OF SPIRIT LED WEIGHT LOSS

SENECA SCHURBON & LEAH LESESNE, MA

DISCLAIMER

We are not doctors, licensed dietitians, or licensed counselors. The information in this book should not be seen as medical, nutritional, or mental health advice and is not intended to take the place of consulting licensed health-care professionals. Check with your doctor, dietitian, counselor, and/or other health professional before implementing any of the suggestions outlined in this book.

Any results stated should be seen as personal testimonies and cannot be guaranteed. The FDA has not evaluated this program for its effectiveness with weight loss.

Acknowledgements

Special thanks to the Rabbit Holers, who are always game for experiments. You kept us moving forward with the writing, let us into your emotional process, and in many ways drove the content of this book.

CONTENTS

INTRODUCTION

Welcome to the no-diet, no-exercise, weight-loss program! We are here to interrupt your usual dieting track record. You know the one:

- Start crazy diet
- Lose some weight
- Stop crazy diet because it's well, crazy and not sustainable
- Gain weight back
- Find another crazy diet, or worse, switch to so-called lifestyle eating because you really believe you can go without _____ for the rest of your life
- Gain weight back, plus some

Just stop already. It's been proven over and over that diets don't work—so much so that they are being rebranded as "healthy lifestyles," yet the focus is still some kind of restriction and losing weight. Because of biology, the more you try, the harder it becomes to lose weight, and typically a lack of will power is blamed. But it's not you that's the failure; it's the premise of the diet industry that you can fight your biology and actually win.

You may have suspected some hidden reasons why you have such a hard time with weight loss. Maybe you blame your metabolism, your thyroid, hormones, or other mysterious factors. The truth is, so much more is going on than calories in, calories out. Many factors within the body and mind influence your weight. This thirty-day plan addresses them one by one.

If you need to drop ten pounds by Saturday to fit into a dress, this is not the book for you. But you'll want to keep reading if any of the following apply:

- You are done with insanity workouts (yes, they are actually named that)
- You are done excluding food groups
- You are done not being able to have a normal meal with people
- You have a bit of patience for healing

The premise of our program is that, each day, you'll spend a few minutes speaking from your spirit to your body. Each day has a different topic with a short explanation of how and why it contributes to your weight, followed by an example of what you can say to your body to initiate healing.

We don't give you any rules about food although as a result of speaking to your body, your eating will probably shift a bit. The people who have already used our program have reported fewer cravings, less hunger, and eating better quality food.

We know that talking to yourself might have a stigma of craziness. But be honest, you've done crazier things to lose weight, right?

You may be familiar with speaking positive declarations over yourself. This is similar, but instead of just speaking some truth and calling it done, we're working on building the lines of communication between your spirit, soul, and body so that you gain a new awareness of ongoing conversation and understanding within yourself.

The best part? Since you don't need any special food, such as so-called meal replacement shakes, workout contraptions, or other involved gadgets, you can start today!

Some Testimonies from those that have Already Tried the Program

"I'm down two pounds in thirty days, and I have a better attitude toward my body. I've begun a needful process of making peace with and partnering with my body."
-Jane I.

"I lost five pounds in thirty days. Looking at food differently has been the biggest difference. My body isn't craving junk food, and because I'm feeling better, I'm walking more, which I love to do."
-Sue B.

"I'm loving my body more and am very encouraged to keep doing the body coaching."
-Cheryl L.

"I lost seven pounds, and I purposely was not dieting! I've noticed a significant difference in the past couple weeks in the ability for my spirit to rise above my emotions/soul and implement positive mindsets. This is HUGE for me!"
-Veronica M.

"This is the first time the scales have gone in a negative direction in years. I have tried a few diets, but the scales never budged. Down 6.4 pounds in a little over three weeks!"
-Rachel S.

"After I started Body Coaching, people commented on my physical appearance, being pretty and looking good. That normally doesn't happen. I was more aware of feeling full, rather than hungry. In the past I ate regardless, and only because my mind automatically thinks I should be eating. Some days I while I was Body Coaching, I wasn't sure what I ate, as my mind was not preoccupied with food. I chose foods quite often that wouldn't make me feel crummy."
– Tammy T.

BODY COACHING

HOW WE GOT HERE
– Seneca –

My eating initially went downhill at age fifteen. I came home one day, and the rest of my family was eating early. They looked surprised to see me. I asked, "Where's mine?" My mom stood up and gave me her food. That was the moment when it sank in that we didn't have enough to eat. While I knew before that we had money problems, this was my first unavoidable evidence.

Our way of life and family business had been disrupted, and in my mind, it was my fault. In my usual over-dramatic teenage fashion, I took full responsibility and stopped eating. I wasn't going to contribute to the problem any more than I already had.

Oh, I would eat if I was around friends who were eating cookies and offered me one, or I'd drink a soda with them. Sugar would be the only thing I'd consume in four days. *Hello, hypoglycemia!*

I'd come home from school, go fishing until dark, and only eat if there was enough. I got lots of compliments on my weight loss; I was the girl on the fish-and-berry diet.

Fast-forward ten years. My interest in natural health and nutrition morphed into orthorexia, an obsession with eating only healthy food. This eating disorder is very sneaky because you can justify everything you're doing. For me, this was a constant state of meal planning, meal prep, cleaning up, gardening to grow fresh and organic foods, and then shopping for the next round of meals. This time-consuming process didn't leave room for a whole lot of life left after that.

When I finally woke up and realized I had a problem, I knew I had to give up control. That was when my husband learned to cook. I did a lot of *Fear Factor* style eating, and my friends put up with texts like "Oh my gosh, I just ate a banana!" (Fructose and high-glycemic foods were my big evil.) I settled into a "living by faith with food" lifestyle where I didn't eat unless somebody fed me, and I would eat whatever it was gratefully. It took care of my teenage lack issue as well as my need to control food.

I didn't exactly waste away. Over several years of this, I put on thirty pounds. And since I was out of the kitchen, I started two businesses and wrote some books, all while working full time.

I felt that the thirty pounds were an okay trade off for all I had gained as far as getting my life back as well as the good I was accomplishing for others. Yet I wondered, *At what point do I find a healthy balance?*

I didn't have the time to diet; I didn't want to focus on that nor did I want to lose my blessing of those that fed me. I also didn't want to start telling them how to better take care of me. I was praying for a solution.

Enter the Solution

The solution came in the least expected way. In my business, Freedom Flowers, we test and develop new flower essences (which are not the same as essential oils). They are primarily used for emotional healing, but we were on the trail of something to help the spirit.

If you can strengthen the spirit so that it leads your body and soul, it accelerates the healing process for both. We were looking for the fast track for difficult conditions that typically take years of therapy.

I put together a blend of everything I could think of to help the spirit, and we tested it. Approximately two people had good results; the rest of us had horrible experiences. I dropped out of testing pretty quickly and pulled the plug on the experiment.

Leah and I were looking over our compiled data, trying to figure out where to go from here, and she felt like the body and soul were fighting against the spirit. We had products in the blend to aid the spirit, but nothing to ease the threat of the status quo being turned upside down by those radical spirits.

We followed the breadcrumbs to Chrysanthemum. I wasn't growing any, but found some at a local nursery. I felt, however, like it needed to be an older, yellow variety. Leah happened to have it. So we tested Chrysanthemum even though we really didn't know what we were looking for in terms of spirit, soul, and body interaction or if it would even work. But the breadcrumbs led us there.

Interesting Results

During testing, an interesting thing happened, most of us developed insomnia. Leah noticed that she was speaking to herself on those sleepless nights, but it felt different than her normal self-talk and she was able to fall asleep. So the rest of us started instructing our bodies with simple commands, such as, "Go back to sleep; you can do it," or "muscles relax, uncramp, and be peaceful." "Go to sleep and wake up in two hours," or "You don't need to be awake right now; you need to rest to feel good." Within a few nights we all saw instant shifts in our sleep doing this type of self-talk.

Now I have not had these kinds of results before. I have certainly tried speaking to my body, taking authority over issues, and similar commands. But I found it easier to get results on somebody else instead of myself. With all this came a kindness and an understanding. The only commanding was when a negative entity was involved. Instead, the rest was more like coaching along the lines of, "I know you can do it."

I put a note out for anybody taking chrysanthemum to do a dominion check. In other words, check to see if the person had greater dominion over their physical body. They tested this on something they'd had prayer or medical intervention for but that had not yet budged.

A migraine vanished instantly. A twenty-year-old intestinal issue shifted with new awareness. A flu duration shortened. Plantar fasciitis improved and the true cause was revealed. Other participants experienced assorted small wins.

Like any kid with a shiny new toy, I played with it all day long. I felt like some mild food poisoning was coming on. So I told my digestive system that it handles stuff like this like a champ, and it just needed to make a little more stomach acid, I mentally connected a memory of when I felt that happen.(I usually have a stomach like a trash compactor, so none of what I said was a lie).

Then I told my body that it had always been wise in the past, so I granted it permission to push this out either end. (Sorry. Body stuff can be graphic.) I commanded the toxins to be neutralized, had an uncomfortable half-hour, and then all was well.

I had some other physical areas that weren't operating in as much wisdom as I thought my digestive system was. I told my muscles to relax. I told the various groups that pointed to an emotional root of feeling unsupported (not true) that we have more support now than in all the previous years put together and that they didn't need to maintain that holding pattern.

Even if all the support went away, life would not be as hard as it was. I told my body to relax. I told my feet that they had support for walking the weird paths, that they were celebrated for this. The pain left but then popped up elsewhere, which often indicates a spiritual root. I told the spirit to go and told my body parts that if they resisted the devil, he would flee. They didn't have to passively accept everything that comes their way.

I put up a poll just to try to gauge numbers on the dominion-check experiment. Most people said that some (not all) of their physical issues resolved; the second-highest number stated that it just plain worked. The third group said that it worked, but the problem came back. Nobody reported that it didn't work at all.

We also talked about the difference in how we were speaking to ourselves. If we spoke from our spirit, the words and tone were awesomely kind and compassionate. But our soul ordered us around in a bossy, take-charge manner. This new self-talk voice has love in it.

Chrysanthemum with Weight Loss

After we had our fun dealing with our main physical issues, we decided we could probably talk our bodies into losing weight as well. We already had a group of volunteer test subjects to work with. We asked for those who wanted to lose weight but who weren't currently doing anything about it (non-dieters).

We split them into two groups. One group didn't use essences but received body-talk conversation starters every day; the other group used chrysanthemum flower essence and the same conversation starters. The chrysanthemum group averaged a three-pound loss over thirty days; the non-essence group lost an average of .7 pounds over the same time period. The range for both groups was from gaining 3.2 pounds to losing 9 pounds.

As soon as I started writing conversation starters, I knew in my spirit that my snacking was a problem. Other people weren't doing such a bad job of feeding me, but in my uncertainty of my next meal, I was fortifying just in case. I wasn't allowing myself to go hungry, and so I bought some packaged junk food when it was convenient. Interestingly, my conviction was not over my lack of faith, but a genuine concern that snacking was harmful.

How could that be? We're told that snacking is good for weight loss and maintaining blood-sugar levels. I did some research and found my answers. I didn't have to overhaul my diet; I didn't have to turn down meals from those who wanted to help me. I just had to start coaching my body through letting go of snacks and letting go of the weight.

As you walk through the written conversation starters, be sensitive and let your spirit help you find the areas where you are sabotaging your body and your health. These will be different for everyone.

LOSING WEIGHT THE BODY COACHING WAY

As you might have gathered so far, this book is not a diet book. We won't be telling you how or how not to eat or what exercise regimen you need to do. We thought about calling the book, *The No-Diet, No-Exercise, Weight-Loss Miracle*, but that sounded too far-fetched to put on a book cover.

While we do expect that you will see changes in your weight and overall health as you go through the book, we're taking a totally different approach than you are probably accustomed to.

Gaining to Lose

If you are currently dieting, including so-called lifestyle changes, and you stop dieting to do this and eat normally, you will gain weight in the short term. We're wired to maintain weight as a protection against starvation, so when you have a history of food restriction, your metabolism slows and conservation mode begins.

The more you diet, the more your body tries to hold on to your weight; therefore, you have to keep upping the ante and trying new tactics. But you can only cut out so much and only keep up with so many rules. While you might be successful at losing the weight now, you'll need to ask yourself if you want to continue down this road.

It may take time to re-establish balance in your body and mind and begin to drop weight. During that time, you might worry as you watch the scale go up, but in the long term, being free with food is worth it. In this context, *free* means free to eat whatever you want, yet also free from being driven by cravings. You are free to eat three square meals a day, but nothing dire happens if you miss one.

Our intention is not to tell you what or how much to eat. With a healed body and mind, you should be able to self-regulate very nicely. The human body has done so for thousands of years. In the interim, it takes time to do the major repair work that involves so many body systems as well as your mindsets and attitudes. Be patient with yourself and your body. You did not get where you are overnight, nor is this the quick fix that the diet industry so often presents.

Healthy weight loss is a half to two pounds a week. If you lose more than that, I suspect you are losing water and muscle rather than fat. If you lose more than that, it sets off alarm bells in the body, saying "Oh, my gosh! We're wasting away! Put on the brakes!"

Another consideration with dieting is that both of us authors are in professions where we work with emotionally upset, stressed-out people. If you are going through some emotional issues, recovering from some trauma, or living with a lot of stress (and, frankly, who isn't these days?) then the last thing your body needs is the additional stress of deprivation of carbs, calories, good fats, and healthy foods. This will raise cortisol and other stress hormones that work against your efforts, again selling your health down the river for some short-term weight loss.

Spirit, Soul, and Body Working in Harmony

As we touched on earlier, our personal spirits were an integral part of the original body coaching discovery. Our efforts were centered on getting our spirits to a place where they could do what was necessary for our healing.

We believe the proper order is spirit—soul—body, and that our spirits should be leading. Our spirit has a direct line to God and was possibly even pre-programmed to have everything needed for every challenge we would meet in life.

Since engaging our spirits in the body coaching process, the most marked difference is the level of compassion with which it responds to the body and soul. It uses a very understanding tone and seems wise and loving even when it is putting its foot down.

We've noticed this in contrast to prior self-talk that had an edge to it even when we were trying to be self-nurturing.

So why haven't we been hearing from our spirits all this time? Your soul is a bit of a control freak. The more strong-willed or stubborn your personality is, the more that is true, but this still applies in most individuals. Because the soul likes control, it projects that onto the spirit, who is really good at control but not into control for control's sake. Soul doesn't like the idea of giving control to the spirit because:

- It no longer has it,
- What the spirit does, doesn't always make sense, and
- Because the soul assumes that spirit will be just as domineering as the soul and now soul will be on the receiving end.

Your body gets sucked into the whole control debacle because it's an easy target. When so many things in life are beyond your ability to control them, our souls tend to look at the body as a way that they can exert some level of dominance over circumstances. This can manifest in different ways, but being rigid with food is very typical. Control gives us a sense of having power and supremacy in our lives.

Putting Your Spirit in Charge

Putting your spirit in charge has been the challenge for many spiritual healers. Your spirit is non-assertive and has definitely been sidelined by society and our upbringing, even if we consider ourselves spiritual people. The majority of what we consider our spiritual practices are really engaged via the soul.

Our method so far has been to use chrysanthemum essence as it seems to help settle the soul down enough so that your spirit can not only talk but be heard. Once your soul sees how this works and understands that it will not be railroaded, that it still has a place, and that your spirit is for it and not against it, the soul relaxes further. You'll be able to quit using chrysanthemum and still speak from your spirit.

To be honest, I (Seneca) notice a mix of soul and spirit when I'm body coaching. I don't worry about it. We aren't of the mindset that the soul is bad or wrong. Ideally, we want spirit and soul in partnership. We do not want the soul to shut up, but we do want the wisdom of the spirit present and in charge.

The talking points presented in this book are not so much for you to read to yourself *verbatim* but topics for exploration with your spirit. You can read them as is to yourself, but from there, also allow your spirit to personalize it for your situation and address any related issues. As you begin, whether you use chrysanthemum or not, set an intention to speak from your spirit.

Using Flower Essences to Support Your Process

You've already heard about chrysanthemum flower essence and how this came about. I'll (Seneca) back up a bit and explain flower essences in general. They are not the same thing as essential oils; they are water-based, don't smell, and are tasteless in anything except plain water.

They work using the frequencies of flowers to heal rather than by any biochemical means, so they have no drug interactions. We typically use them for emotional healing. Rather than unpack all the nuts and bolts here, I have a free email mini-course on my website if you'd like to learn more:

www.freedom-flowers.com/start-here/

In addition to the chrysanthemum essence that we use for the body coaching, another blend of essences my company makes is called Craving Control.

Craving Control helps foster a healthy mindset and proper motivation and addresses the emotional aspects of stress eating, addiction, and self-medicating. Not only is it helpful with eating disorders, but it is also ideal for anyone who wants to have a healthier relationship with food.

Using flower essences is easy. Four drops go into whatever you're drinking. Typically, we use them throughout the day, although many people experience insomnia when they use chrysanthemum too close to bedtime. It's not necessary to use essences with the body-conversation starters, but it will probably make your process a bit smoother.

If It Works Too Well

As your body begins to move towards health, you might experience what is called a healing crisis. When too many toxins leave your body too quickly, you may experience some of these symptoms:

- Muscle soreness
- Fatigue
- Headaches
- Cold-like symptoms
- Diarrhea
- Acne or rash outbreaks
- Nausea

These symptoms will eventually pass as your body deals with all the junk. Drink lots of water and give yourself time to rest to support your body in this process, and if certain things are contributing to the problem of too-much, too-fast, cut back until the symptoms subside and then ease yourself back into it.

Healing crises are not the norm with flower essences, but can definitely happen. If you are having a rough time since starting an essence, this will hopefully shed a little light.

First, let's remember that, in the natural-health world, the so-called healing crisis is always a good thing. It means the treatment is working, albeit a little too well. Many of you are familiar with cleansing. If you overdo it, you experience a range of nasty symptoms, which simply means that you need to back off a bit and do a little less.

Essences work exactly the same way except you're cleaning out old hurts and baggage that you've been hanging onto that isn't serving you well. It can be painful to see this stuff come to the surface and have your false fronts stripped away.

If it becomes too intense, then stop for a couple days, let things settle, and try again with less frequent doses. The other option is to look at what you're taking and try a different approach with new essences. As you become stronger, you can then come back to the troubling essences later.

TAPPING WHILE YOU TALK
- Leah -

Our bodies store memories of emotion. Have you ever been a in a yoga class and suddenly felt a wave of emotion when you held a certain pose? Or felt butterflies in your stomach, heartbreak in your chest, or had a gut feeling? We all have experiences of feeling emotion in our bodies, but rarely do we acknowledge the lasting impression they can leave.

Fortunately, there are ways to release the body memories of emotion. One tool I use with my clients is tapping through body-meridian points while focusing on a particular issue or emotion.

You may have heard of Emotional Freedom Technique (EFT) or Thought Field Therapy (TFT) tapping. I'm trained in both, but the method I use is my own creation called Captive Thought Therapy (CTT).

Where Captive Thought Therapy differs from other tapping protocols is that we don't just focus on clearing out the negative. We also spend time downloading the good and declaring truth over ourselves.

As you go through the conversation starters in *Body Coaching*, you can add this tapping exercise to help fully engage your body–mind–spirit and help clear out any emotional blocks.

Variations of this exercise are called the Peak Performance Algorithm in TFT and other modalities. In Captive Thought Therapy, I call it the Full Potential Exercise because it's all about living out of our God-given potential, not a performance mentality.

For more on Captive Thought Therapy and how it can help with other emotional issues visit:

www.CaptiveThoughtTherapy.com

Full Potential Exercise

A – E – CB – BH+B(30) – SH

Tap three to five times on each point as you do the Body Coaching from each day's conversation starters or whatever else you know that you need to speak to your body.

When you get to BH+B(30), tap the BH–back of hand point continuously for at least 30 seconds while stepping back and forth or moving your eyes side to side for B–bilateral brain stimulation.

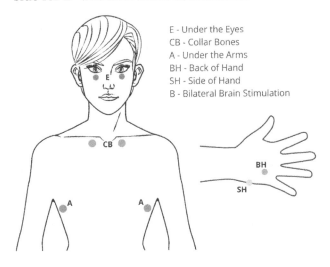

E - Under the Eyes
CB - Collar Bones
A - Under the Arms
BH - Back of Hand
SH - Side of Hand
B - Bilateral Brain Stimulation

Forgiveness Statements

You may find as you read that there is some forgiveness you need to do in addition to the Body Coaching. Another tapping exercise you may find helpful is forgiveness statements.

Forgiving Yourself

As you forgive yourself or your body, tap on the side of your index finger at the nail and repeat the forgiveness statement three times, then tap on the side of your hand three to five times.

Forgiving Others

If you are forgiving another person, tap on the side of your pinky finger at the nail. Repeat the forgiveness statement three times, then tap on the side of your hand.

Forgiving God

You may find that you need to forgive God. Forgiveness is about our resentments, so we aren't saying that God did anything wrong; we're just recognizing the offenses we've held against him and choosing to let them go.

When forgiving God, tap on the side of your middle finger while repeating the forgiveness statement three times, then tap the side of your hand three to five times.

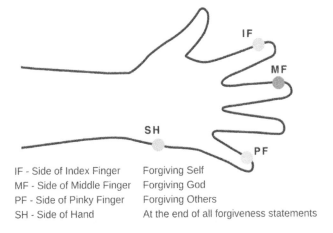

IF - Side of Index Finger   Forgiving Self
MF - Side of Middle Finger   Forgiving God
PF - Side of Pinky Finger   Forgiving Others
SH - Side of Hand   At the end of all forgiveness statements

Sample forgiveness statements:

I forgive myself for bullying my body

I forgive my mom for making negative comments about my weight.

I forgive God for giving me a body that struggles with health issues.

BODY COACHING

LISTENING TO YOUR BODY CLOCK
- Leah -

Your body clock is a powerful timepiece. The meridian clock combined with your circadian rhythm can tell a lot about your physical and emotional health. Throughout the day, body systems are active or resting at different times.

Knowing what systems are active and when can give you insight into what problems you are facing or may face soon. The circadian rhythm is your inner clock that knows to get up when the sun rises and to become sleepy when it sets.

Our modern culture with blackout curtains and bright electronics late at night can mix up our circadian rhythms and leave our bodies a little confused as to when we are supposed to do what.

Finding Your Time Zone

Fortunately, in addition to our circadian rhythms, we also have the internal meridian
clock that keeps our bodies cycling even if we aren't quite sure what time it is.

The meridian clock cycle doesn't change, but if your circadian rhythm is off, your meridian times may be different than those listed here.

By paying attention to your personal meridian cycle and by being mindful of your light exposure in the early morning and evening, you can reset your circadian rhythm to a more natural time.

For each time bracket, you can track both the physical and emotional processes to determine your body clock's time zone. Certain emotions are associated with each meridian where our bodies tend to store a physical memory of those emotions.

Holding meridian points (over clothes is fine) and focusing thought around those emotions can help the body release the memory and relieve the emotional trigger. Often when we release emotional triggers, we also see positive release or healing in the physical as well.

These point holding exercises are related to the tapping work we discussed in the last chapter and are also a component of Captive Thought Therapy.

The Body Clock Meridians

5-7 a.m. | Large Intestine

Physical: This is a great time to wake up, drink water, and let your bowels start moving. When your colon is empty, you'll have an easier time digesting your breakfast without feeling sluggish.

Emotional: Some negative emotions that you may find yourself dealing with during this time are perfectionism, self-hatred, or yearning. If you notice yourself feeling any of those holding one hand over your large intestine (right over your belly button) and your other hand on your forehead while you think about the emotion you are feeling can help the emotion move on faster.

7-9 a.m. | Stomach

Physical: While your stomach is engaged, this is the perfect time to eat a nutritious breakfast.

Emotional: Some negative emotions that you may find yourself dealing with during this time are worry, over-responsibility, or hopelessness. If you notice yourself feeling any of those holding one hand over your stomach (just below your rib cage) and your other hand on your forehead while you think about the emotion you are feeling can help the emotion move on faster.

9-11 a.m. | Spleen

Physical: Your metabolism is at a peak during this meridian, and you're more mentally sharp to get work done.

Emotional: Some negative emotions that you may find yourself dealing with during this time are apathy, entitlement, or self-consciousness. If you notice yourself feeling any of those holding one hand over your spleen (lower left side of rib cage) and your other hand on your forehead while you think about the emotion you are feeling can help the emotion move on faster.

11 a.m. -1 p.m. | Heart

Physical: This is a great time to eat heart-healthy foods and engage socially.

Emotional: Some negative emotions that you may find yourself dealing with during this time are insecurity, abandonment, or unforgiveness. If you notice yourself feeling any of those touching your fingertips over your heart (center of the chest) and holding your other hand on your forehead while you think about the emotion you are feeling can help the emotion move on faster.

1-3 p.m. | Small Intestine

Physical: As your body is digesting lunch, this is a good time to get back to work.

Emotional: Some negative emotions that you may find yourself dealing with during this time are denial, vulnerability, or lack of emotion. If you notice yourself feeling any of those holding one hand over your small intestine (right over your belly button) and your other hand on your forehead while you think about the emotion you are feeling can help the emotion move on faster.

3-5 p.m. | Bladder

Physical: Drink plenty of water to support your body in natural detoxing processes. Read, finish up work, and begin to let your mind unwind for the day.

Emotional: Some negative emotions that you may find yourself dealing with during this time are fear, dread, or bad memories. If you notice yourself feeling any of those holding one hand over your bladder (lower abdomen) and your other hand on your forehead while you think about the emotion you are feeling can help the emotion move on faster.

5-7 p.m.| Kidney

Physical: Eat dinner to replenish your energy and to keep your kidneys from working too hard.

Emotional: Some negative emotions that you may find yourself dealing with during this time are shame, timidity, or unworthiness. If you notice yourself feeling any of those holding one hand over your kidneys (either side of your lower back) and your other hand on your forehead while you think about the emotion you are feeling can help the emotion move on faster.

7-9 p.m. | Reproductive Organs

Physical: This is a great time for intimacy or to take a relaxing bath to promote circulation.

Emotional: Some negative emotions that you may find yourself dealing with during this time are jealousy, muddled thoughts and feelings, or love unreturned. If you notice yourself feeling any of those holding one hand over your pelvis (lower abdomen) and your other hand on your forehead while you think about the emotion you are feeling can help the emotion move on faster.

9-11 p.m. | Endocrine

Physical: Avoid eating after this time in the evening and allow your body to prepare for sleep by regulating temperature and metabolism.

Emotional: Some negative emotions that you may find yourself dealing with during this time are paranoia, depletion, or nightmares. If you notice yourself feeling any of those holding one hand over your thyroid (right over your throat) and your other hand on your forehead while you think about the emotion you are feeling can help the emotion move on faster.

11 p.m. -1 a.m. | Gallbladder

Physical: Allow your body to sleep and engage in regenerative processes.

Emotional: Some negative emotions that you may find yourself dealing with during this time are bitterness, resentment, or trouble forgiving. If you notice yourself feeling any of those holding one hand over your gallbladder (lower right side of your ribcage) and your other hand on your forehead while you think about the emotion you are feeling can help the emotion move on faster. You may also need to declare your decision to forgive someone. See the forgiveness tapping in the previous chapter for some extra help forgiving.

1-3 a.m. | Liver

Physical: Your body should be sleeping deeply and performing detoxing processes. If you wake up frequently during this time, you may be putting too much of a toxic load on your body, especially alcohol.

Emotional: Some negative emotions that you may find yourself dealing with during this time are depression, anger, or powerlessness. If you notice yourself feeling any of those holding one hand over your liver (lower right side of your rib cage) and your other hand on your forehead while you think about the emotion can help it clear faster.

3-5 a.m. | Lung

Physical: These are the final stages of sleep. Your body should be feeling restored and well rested.

Emotional: Some negative emotions that you may find yourself dealing with during this time are grief, loneliness, or betrayal. If you notice yourself feeling any of those holding one hand over your lung (either side of chest just in front of armpit) and your other hand on your forehead while you think about the emotion you are feeling can help the emotion move on faster.

Getting Back in Rhythm

Once you've discovered the time zone of your body clock, you may realize that your meridian clock keeps being disrupted at times. If you keep waking up at the same time in the middle of the night or if you feel sudden fatigue during the same time every day, the meridian clock can help you figure out what is causing the disruption.

Paying attention to your meridian body clock can also help you notice when you might be dealing with physical problems that you hadn't realized were bothering you. Dealing with those issues early on can minimize the overall damage to your health.

If part of your struggle is that the lack of light tricks your body during the winter or when using black-out curtains, a sunrise alarm clock can help give your body a natural wake-up cue.

Using an app for your phone or a similar program on your computer that's designed to help lessen your exposure to blue light in the evenings can also help improve sleep. Alternatively, you could try putting away all electronics for a few hours before bedtime.

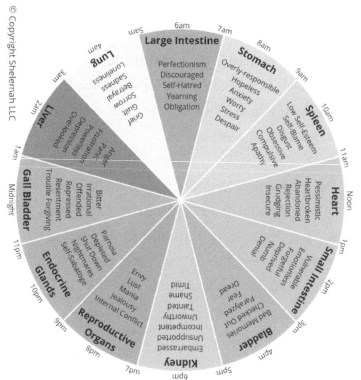

Body Meridian Clock of Emotions

HOW TO USE THIS BOOK

To maximize the effectiveness of the book, we recommend using the Body Coaching Program from Seneca's site at www.freedom-flowers.com/body-coaching-weight-loss-program. With the program, you'll receive the following supports for your journey:

- Email reminders of the daily conversation starters
- Membership in an exclusive Facebook group and the support of others doing Body Coaching
- A bottle of Chrysanthemum flower essence, and
- A bottle of Craving Control flower essence blend

You do not need to the program to use the book and do Body Coaching, but we do recommend having some form of support and community as you go through the book.

Best Practices as You Read

Set an intention that when you speak to your body, you will speak from your spirit. Don't worry about whether you're doing it right or not. It's normal to have your soul in the mix as you approach this from an academic standpoint of reading a book.

Every day, you'll spend a few minutes doing one of the Conversation Starters, and you can tap along with it. Participating in meaningfully engaged talking when first learning to tap might be challenging, so you might practice the tapping algorithm first or talk with no tapping and then combine the two.

The Conversation Starters on each day are not merely for you to read to yourself but are examples of conversations to start with your body. You might begin by reading them verbatim but also give a little thought to your unique situation, how to apply the points personally, and speak in your own words.

Each day has a space for you to journal other aspects of conversation that come to mind. Some of the days will resonate with you more than others, and you'll begin to see how to apply different ones throughout the day.

- If there are people around, it's okay to say the Conversation Starters silently to yourself.

- If you use flower essences, add them to whatever you drink throughout the day.

- Make a mental note of times of the day when you struggle physically or become tired or times at night when you wake up. Use the chapter, *Listening to Your Body Clock*, on page 33 to address those issues.

- Fight the urge to go back to the familiar diet and exercise attempts to lose weight. If you find yourself naturally making shifts while going through the book, that's great! But don't impose new regimes on yourself right now.

BODY COACHING

A LOVE LETTER FROM YOUR BODY

Dear Soul,

We have been through some tough times together. I think you might need to hear that no matter what, I'm always on your side.

I have garnered you attention at times and not always the right kind, if you get my drift. You've been made to suffer because of how I looked. From lustful advances to body shaming ridicule, you, my soul, have felt it deep in your core. At times, you felt betrayed by me, but I want you to know that these things were neither of our faults. It says so much more about our perpetrators than it does about us. All of the words spoken about how we look—let them fall to the ground right now. There is so much more to us!

I use everything you give me. I'm a master at taking the little and allocating to the very most important thing we need at any given time. At times, I've been forced to make some hard decisions when I didn't have enough.

You might have been in a hard place yourself financially, or you might have been dieting, fasting, or dealing with an eating disorder. During those times, I did what I had to do to keep us going. I might still suffer from some PTSD from that, so your patience and love is appreciated. As we open up communication, I'll try to trust you. Please forgive me for when I've been fearful and attempted to conserve energy by staying heavy.

Soul, I know that, at times, your pain was beyond your ability to cope. Cutting was a way out of feeling numb or a way to release internal pain on the outside. Substances like food, alcohol, drugs, or other alternatives helped you face the things that you couldn't bear. I was with you through it all, holding on to your life for you until you grew strong enough to hold on for yourself. I'm glad you're still here. I never stopped loving you.

You might see me as natural, purely physical, but that's shortsighted. I'm not the same as you, soul, but

I have recorded every emotional thing you've ever been through. I probably know more about you than you know about yourself. I understand how it affected you because it affected me too. We are inexplicably connected, and the lines between us aren't clear. I wouldn't have it any other way. I love being a part of you. I love partnering with you in all that we do. Our collaboration makes us a force for good in this world!

Our history—the good, the bad, and the ugly—has made us who we are. We are wiser for our mistakes, stronger from our breakdowns, and more beautiful than ever for our raw reality.

Do you understand that I know all your junk and love you all the more for it? Do you understand that my heart beats for you? I am here for you.

Love,
Your Body

BODY COACHING

DAY 1 BODY, I'M SORRY

We've said or done so many negative things to ourselves because we were unhappy with our weight. Fooling the body into thinking it's starving by disallowing fat or carbohydrates can cause physical trauma. And calling ourselves fat adds further emotional trauma that your body feels as well. Add the constant battles over the years, and you can understand why your body might react to this as "here we go again." It might help to state your new intentions up front to repair the rift. Only you know your history, so don't be afraid to go deep today.

Conversation Starters:

Body, I'm sorry for how I've treated you in the past, for being impatient with you, for becoming frustrated when you didn't or couldn't do what I wanted, for depriving you, punishing you, or in any way fighting against you as if we weren't on the same team.

Body, this time is different. I'm not going to bully you. I'm going to coach you lovingly like the friend I should have been to you all along. I want to be fully in tune with what you need and with what makes you feel good. Let's work together on this health thing!

Continue the Conversation:

Take this space to journal out any other conversations you know you need to have with your body about the day's topic.

DAY 2 LOW METABOLISM

If you have a track record of dieting, including so-called lifestyle eating, you might have a damaged metabolism. When you restrict your eating in any way, including calorie counting, low carb, Paleo, or anything else, your body will attempt to defend its fat-mass set point, whether high or low, over the long term by increasing hunger and reducing metabolic rate.

One way of testing this is to take your temperature in the morning before you get up and become active. The normal body temperature is 98.6° although that varies. If you are lower than 98.0°, your metabolism has definitely taken a hit. Sometimes this can indicate hypothyroidism, but if that condition hasn't shown up on medical tests, a low metabolic rate might be the culprit.

Conversation Starters:

Body, there is enough. I know, in the past, there might not have been enough because of resources or because I hurt you with restrictive diets. But I promise that from now on, if you need food, you will get it.

We live in a country abundant with food; there's no reason to fear that we'll starve. When we do eat, we can eat just what we need and what we actually enjoy. We don't need to stuff ourselves to the point of not enjoying what we ate so that we feel sick.

Body, it's okay to raise that metabolic rate. If you do, we'll be less likely to get sick; we'll sleep deeper, process toxins more efficiently, and have more energy.

You have a lot of safeguards built in to protect me against famine, but that's not a threat right now.

Even if we become a little busy and don't eat on time, we are not going to starve. Your natural design is to be lean and to bring up that metabolic rate.

Let's forget every instance of the past when you felt you needed to hold on to fat. Now restore to your original setting and start fresh. We don't need to hoard the fat to survive. We are safe in abundance.

Continue the Conversation:

Take this space to journal out any other conversations you know you need to have with your body about the day's topic.

BODY COACHING

DAY 3 ORIGINAL BLUEPRINT

Our bodies are amazing creations. We have so many systems in place to keep us up and running even when we have some dysfunction. We need to look holistically at the entire package when moving back toward balance rather than directing all our attention toward one issue. The endocrine system alone is a great example as every gland interacts with each other: the thyroid, adrenals, pancreas, ovaries in women, and testes in men. When one area goes off track, your body develops a sort of work-around solution.

Conversation Starters:

Body, you're doing a great job. You have so many systems and processes working together. Let's look at the original blueprint and move back toward that. All the different functions have to move slowly back toward their original design because, when one gets out of sync, others adjust to compensate. So all systems listen up: let's agree together right now to cooperate and align for our full potential.

Continue the Conversation:

Take this space to journal out any other conversations you know you need to have with your body about the day's topic.

DAY 4 WHAT HAPPENED WHEN THE WEIGHT GAIN STARTED?

Promoting healing often all stems back to what was going on when the pain started. The same can be true for weight loss. Several years ago, I (Leah) worked in a group home for girls who had come out of sex trafficking. The home was a toxic environment with really dangerous leadership and an ultimately high-stress and unsafe working environment. I ended up living off peanut-butter-and-jelly sandwiches and Cherry Coke for several months because we barely had a chance to eat while working.

Eventually I had to quit because my physical safety was being threatened on a daily basis, and the staff above me was not taking reasonable precautions to ensure my safety. I gained about ten pounds from the stress and poor diet during that season, not to mention suffering from adrenal fatigue due to being in constant fight-or-flight mode. Part of losing weight for me has been processing with my body about that traumatic season and reminding myself that I am safe now.

Think back to when you really put on the weight. What was going on in your life at the time?

Conversation Starters:

Body, we've been through some tough times together. You handled those traumatic seasons the best you knew how, and I'm glad we made it through the storm. I'm sorry for how I didn't feed you well and didn't take proper care of you in that season. I was just doing the best I could to survive too.

But, body, we are in a safe place now. We can let go of all the extra baggage we picked up in that season. We can grieve the losses without losing our health too.

Continue the Conversation:

Take this space to journal out any other conversations you know you need to have with your body about the day's topic.

BODY COACHING

DAY 5 CRAVINGS AND DOPAMINE ADDICTION

We talked about the metabolism and body-fat set point, which works through hunger and fullness levels and increasing or decreasing the metabolism as needed. Just by modifying hunger and metabolism, the body can constantly ensure that calories in equal calories out so that body weight stays stable.

When your body is low on nutrients, you feel hungry and eat more. When you're full of nutrients, you eat less. Your body should constantly modify your eating behavior according to your biological need. It sounds simple except that's not all there is to weight.

One monkey wrench in this mix can be our neurological response to rewarding food. When you eat to release dopamine or to feed an addiction, your neurological function is running the show, and this is independent of what your metabolism is trying to accomplish.[1] This causes you to lose touch with the signals from your body fat set-point system.

As a result of eating to give yourself neurological pleasure, you become numb to the signals telling you to stop eating and instead start listening to your brain's cravings for more pleasure, which leads you to eat more than you need. This is actually why junk food is bad—not so much because of empty calories but because it so critically undermines your ability to regulate your eating.

Conversation Starters:

Body, we might have to learn to say no to some cravings. Brain, you might have been wired to crave food that isn't good for us. So brain, don't freak out if we tell you no. We love you, and we want what's best for you. We have to break the unhealthy patterns that make us think we feel good when we eat junk.

Over time, you'll start to crave food that actually is healthy, and then we all can work together to really enjoy the things we eat. Brain, try to get back in touch with the metabolism so that we eat what we need to when we need to, not because we need a fix. I speak peace and balance to all the neurotransmitters.

Continue the Conversation:

Take this space to journal out any other conversations you know you need to have with your body about the day's topic.

BODY COACHING

DAY 6 EMOTIONAL STATES WHILE EATING

Our emotional state when we eat plays a huge role in how our bodies are able to absorb the nutrients in our food and handle the digestion process smoothly. In Dr. Caroline Leaf's book, *Think and Eat Yourself Smart*, she talks about how even eating healthy foods can damage our bodies when we are in heightened emotional states that do not allow us to digest the food properly and benefit from its nutrients.[2]

If you've relied on food to comfort yourself or forced yourself to eat when you are upset because you feel like you shouldn't miss a meal, you might find that talking to your body about how you're feeling and calming yourself down before you try to eat anything will be much better for your body and your overall wellbeing.

Conversation Starters:

Body, soul, listen up. I know, in the past, we've eaten to cope with our emotions or even just because we felt like we were supposed to eat at a certain time even if we didn't feel like it; but I realize now that eating when we're angry, stressed, or dealing with any form of a negative emotion, actually hurts us more than helps us.

Digestive tract, I'm sorry I expected you to just be able to handle food regardless of our emotional state. I'll work on paying better attention to how we're feeling before we eat and take time to feel better before eating when necessary.

Continue the Conversation:

Take this space to journal out any other conversations you know you need to have with your body about the day's topic.

BODY COACHING

DAY 7 EATING RELIGIOUSLY

I'm (Seneca) keenly aware now how much food idealists are similar to religious denominations. They all have their narrow little focus, the things that they vilify, and they will adamantly insist that their way is the best. These groups include the Paleo people, the low-carb fanatics, the Keto dieters, the vegans, and others. The one thing that they have in common is that they all shun something. And there's merit in all of it, but all of them are missing a piece—or peace.

Does this sound familiar?

"Bless me, trainer, for I have sinned. It's been one day since my last confession."
"One day?"
"Yes, well, I . . . this is hard . . . I . . . oh, I'm so ashamed."
"What is it, my child?"
"Yesterday, at lunch, I ate food that tasted good—and I enjoyed it. There were carbs and everything."
"I see," the trainer answers solemnly. "That *is* bad. Are you repentant?"

"I am! I am! I knew it was wrong, and I am determined to turn away from these sins. But it gets worse."

"Go on."

"When I weighed myself this morning, I had gained 1.3 pounds."

A barely audible gasp is heard across the treadmill.

"I see. Do a kale, cod-liver oil, wheatgrass, spirulina, superfood, alkaline, detox cleanse for the next two weeks followed by thrice daily coffee enemas and steel-wool purification baths for another five days."

"Is that all it will take to purge the evil from my heart . . . and colon?"

"It's a start. Go and sin no more."

-Dr. Steve Prentice in *Wrecked*

Conversation Starters:

Body, I'm sorry for how I might have held onto a legalistic or religious mindset and how that has hurt you. I release that dietary dogma. We don't need to be vegan, vegetarian, meatatarian, Whole 30, Paleo, keto, or any other specific diet approved. We need to be healthy, and we're going to be our healthiest when we are living from a place of love and grace toward ourself instead of any set of rules.

Continue the Conversation:

Take this space to journal out any other conversations you know you need to have with your body about the day's topic.

DAY 8 AVOIDING SNACKS

Today we're not just talking but beginning to listen to how our body feels after meals. Check back a couple hours later to get a read on your hunger and energy levels after each specific meal. You should be running strong hours later if you ate foods that work with your particular biochemistry.

If you need to snack, you might need to tweak your macronutrient ratio (fat, protein, and carbs) so that you make it to the next meal hungry but not famished. This is not a one-size-fits-all plan; some people need more carbs than others while some need more protein. If you're hungry, and you have a couple hours to go until the next meal, eat a snack!

One of the reasons why we want to eat enough so that we don't need to snack is to help your digestive system. Your nervous system consists of the parasympathetic and the sympathetic. The sympathetic mode is fight or flight and lesser forms of chronic stress. We're in parasympathetic mode when we feel safe, when we breathe deeply, and when we feel connected to others, such as at a sit-down meal with your family and friends. In parasympathetic mode, we can digest food properly.[3]

When you snack on the go, you are in sympathetic mode, which cheats your body of nutrients and can create leaky gut, leading to food sensitivities.[4] Your gut can also repair itself if it's allowed to go at least six hours without eating more food.[5]

Your brain and your gut both want satiety, which is that fullness that only comes from a good meal. Meal times were also traditionally a mini-event with family and/or friends and blessings and gratitude. This is a great way to engage the parasympathetic nervous system and switch on digestion, but you can talk to your body when that isn't practical.

We've also been taught that we should eat frequently to keep our metabolism up and to keep our blood-sugar levels stable. If you look through a medical textbook on hypoglycemia, you'll see the recommendation to eat five to six small meals or healthy snacks per day as fortification. What the diet gurus haven't told you is that this is a stop-gap measure to carry you through. You should gradually transition to three meals per day to stabilize your body.

For a period of time, you are also burning up the fuel from your most recent meal. If you are eating every two to three hours, you will never burn from your fat stores.[6] As your body adjusts to eating less frequently throughout the day, it also transitions from only burning the last thing you ate to getting into your fat reserves. Experts are divided at how long after your last meal this happens, and this also seems to take less time once you've gotten into a rhythm of breaks between eating. This transition can take a while but once you are there, your insulin levels will remain stable, and your body will burn fat as its norm.

If you are used to eating throughout the day and you are prone to waking up at night, you might be suffering from stress exhaustion or low-blood sugar. When under stress, the adrenals go looking for energy. Their main go to is the pancreas where stress generates cravings to create energy for the adrenals. Most people react either by eating multiple small meals or by frequent snacking.

If you train your body by feeding it every couple of hours, it learns to only burn that quick fuel instead of body fat, which burns long and slow. When it runs out of fuel in the middle of the night, you don't sleep well.[7]

Conversation Starters:

Body, we're moving away from grazing, but we're still going to eat plenty. We need you to burn fat and keep blood-sugar levels stable as we transition.

At mealtime:

Nervous system, it's time for the parasympathetic to be in charge. We are going to slow down, be present, and enjoy our meal. Digestive system, let's pull all the nourishment we can out of this food.

Before bed:

Body, you need to burn fat for fuel tonight, and let me sleep. Don't wake me up because you think you need some sugar. You have enough in the reserves to serve all systems of the body. Don't freak out because you don't have the easy, fast-burning option. Let's also do some gut-repair work tonight and every night.

Continue the Conversation:

Take this space to journal out any other conversations you know you need to have with your body about the day's topic.

BODY COACHING

DAY 9 HEALTHY IDENTITY

What we believe about ourselves may be the most powerful factor in our health. If you believe you are an unhealthy person that will always be unhealthy, it's going to be very hard for your body to fight you on that.

A good way to identify false identities that you've been claiming is to think about if you would believe those things to be true about others. If you believe others can grow in health and overcome weight loss struggles, why don't you believe that for yourself?

Shame is always tied to identity. So anywhere you are feeling ashamed is another good place to look for a false belief about yourself. When you find those places of false belief, recognize them as such and begin to consciously disavow that belief and actively choose to believe the truth.

Think about what you would say to a dear friend that was struggling to believe positive things about themselves. Your body is that friend, and it needs to hear all the kind, truthful things about itself that it can.

Conversation Starters:

Body, I'm sorry for the times I haven't thought of us as a healthy person. When I've set the bar low and claimed an identity of unhealthy. It may have been through jokes at my own expense because I was embarrassed, but I realize those jokes hurt you.

Body, we are a healthy person. We might not fully be there yet in expressing that identity, but that's where we are headed. It's okay to be in process and to live out what we know to be our true self even if others don't see it yet.

Continue the Conversation:

Take this space to journal out any other conversations you know you need to have with your body about the day's topic.

BODY COACHING

DAY 10 LEPTIN

A lie is floating around that fat people are fat because they eat too much and aren't fit. As you've probably noticed, so many more factors affect weight than calories in, calories out. I (Seneca) eat more than many obese people, yet I don't weigh anywhere near what they weigh. I walk eight miles a day, yet some tubby people beat my step count every day.

If you are under eating, your metabolism will not perform as it should, so this talking point is not for everyone. If you are truly overeating out of hunger, leptin resistance could be an issue. Leptin is a hormone in your bloodstream that signals your hypothalamus that you've had enough food. If you're overweight, you have plenty of leptin, but your receptors aren't picking it up so it signals your brain that you're starving.[8] That can mean hunger except when you physically have no place to put more food.

Conversation Starters:

Body, you might not be picking up the signal that we have enough food. You're going to need to trust me until we can help the brain receive the proper leptin levels.

Brain, you need to try to reconnect with the true levels in the bloodstream. Triglycerides, come down, please.

Body, do whatever you can to decrease inflammation. I know I might have been feeding the problem, and I apologize. I was following my biology.

Leptin, you are awesome. You do me so much good in so many ways—my heart, my immune system, my bones, and fertility—so the last thing I want to do is to run you too low by under eating. But we might need to rely on other body cues until the brain starts tracking with you again. So stay steady, please.

Body, some foods are metabolically toxic and stored in your tissues. These are causing the brain not to receive the signal about how much leptin is in the blood. We need you to direct some energy to purging those toxic stores a little at a time.

Continue the Conversation:

Take this space to journal out any other conversations you know you need to have with your body about the day's topic.

BODY COACHING

DAY 11 IMMUNE SYSTEM

Much as you don't feel like doing anything other than lying around when you are sick, your body doesn't have much energy to give to anything other than getting you well. If you've been fighting any kind of cold, flu, seasonal allergies, or other illness while going through this book, you may not be too surprised if your body just isn't very interested right now. You can still benefit from talking to your body and encouraging it; you just may not see it respond to what you're talking about until it has more energy to do so.

While your immune system needs to deal with real health threats, such as viruses and bacteria, you may also be fighting autoimmune responses. When your immune system forgets who's friend and who's foe, you can end up exhausted as your body fights against itself. It's easy to become frustrated with your immune system for responding this way, but it's all the more important to speak gently to your immune system and encourage it to remember who you are and how to identify yourself.

Conversation Starters:

Body, I know our conversations have been focused on weight loss, but immune system I want to make sure you know I see you. I so appreciate the hard work you do to keep us healthy. I know talking about weight loss when you're battling bacteria or viruses for us can feel really trivial, but ultimately as we lose weight, you will be better equipped to function more efficiently.

Body, you have permission to prioritize immune system issues until we are at a healthy place to move forward with weight loss. And immune system, you have permission to use the resources you need to make us feel better.

Immune system, I also want to make sure you know that it's okay to rest. You may have gone into a panic at times and started attacking things that were not threats. I release you from having to fight any autoimmune battles. Even if you've forgotten, all you need to know about recognizing what is actually a healthy part of us and what is a threat is deep within our DNA.

Continue the Conversation:

Take this space to journal out any other conversations you know you need to have with your body about the day's topic.

BODY COACHING

DAY 12 SLEEP

Lots of studies have been done correlating poor sleep with weight gain. If you don't sleep well, you'll have trouble losing weight, no matter how well you eat. Sleep debt tends to deregulate the appetite and causes us to eat the types of foods that give us that neuro-high. We also may not move around as much due to fatigue.

If you find yourself waking up around the same time every night, check the *Listening to Your Body Clock* chapter on page 33 for more insight on the physical and emotional issues that might be at play. This will help you further discern what you need to talk to your body about.

Conversation Starters:

Body, I know sleep hasn't always been a priority like it should be. We might have even carried a badge of pride that we don't need that much sleep. But we really do need sleep to feel our best. I give you permission to rest, to sleep deeply. Whatever worries we have can wait till we are well rested to face them.

Body, I know, at times, you've felt confused about when we're supposed to sleep. I apologize for ways I've caused that confusion with caffeine and disrupting our circadian rhythm. Body, you need to learn what artificial light is and disregard it as a time clock.

Digestive tract, we need the proper amount of serotonin for the pineal to convert to melatonin at the right time. You know how and when to sleep. You were made to be an expert at restful sleep. I'm sorry for how I've tried to silence you when you've told me it's time to sleep. I promise to do better at listening to you.

Continue the Conversation:

Take this space to journal out any other conversations you know you need to have with your body about the day's topic.

BODY COACHING

DAY 13 MEDICATIONS

Many medications have side effects that include weight gain or water retention. Some make us tired so that we move around less. Over time, some may even harm other body systems out of concern or in attempts to heal the original ones. DO NOT read this as a command to go off your medication, but feel free to speak to the condition that causes you to need the medicine.

In time, you might be able to work with your doctor on decreasing your medication or eliminating it completely. Additionally, the Original Design talking point from Day 3 might need to be a staple for you.

Conversation Starters:

Body, I'm sorry for how the medications we've taken from time to time may have helped one part of you but hurt another. I didn't mean to hurt that other part of you; I just really wanted the part I was trying to help to feel better.

Parts that have been hurt, you have permission to heal. I speak covering and protection over you from any way the medications we need to take might try to harm you.

Body, I know some medications might have tricked you into thinking we needed to hold on to extra water. You have permission to let go of the extra water. I trust you to know how much water we need. And the same goes for anything else extra. If we need more, we can get it. We don't have to carry it around all the time.

Continue the Conversation:

Take this space to journal out any other conversations you know you need to have with your body about the day's topic.

BODY COACHING

DAY 14 HYDRATION

Staying well hydrated is very important for every system in the body to function well. Name a body system; it needs water. Our bodies are made up of about 60 percent water, yet about 75 percent of Americans are chronically dehydrated.[9,10] So it's no wonder that our bodies might be living under a scarcity mentality when it comes to H2O.

Part of the solution is, of course, to be more mindful about drinking enough water every day so that our bodies don't need to hoard water. But if you've already been staying hydrated, your body might just need some assurance that a shortage isn't coming and that it's ok to release the extra water.

Conversation Starters:

Body, I know I talked to you yesterday about holding on to extra water from medications, but I also need to apologize. I've not always done the best job of keeping you hydrated.

Body, I'm sorry for how I've taught you scarcity with water. You don't have to hold onto extra water for fear there won't be more. I promise to pay better attention to you and make sure you get the water you need before we feel overwhelmingly thirsty.

Kidneys, listen up. You're the gatekeepers of all this water. It's time to let those gates open and let go of any extra water we've held on to.[11]

Bladder, that might mean you're going to have to work harder than you have in the past. But you were made for this. You have permission to increase capacity as needed, but you can also count on me to give you enough bathroom breaks to accommodate our increased water intake.

Continue the Conversation:

Take this space to journal out any other conversations you know you need to have with your body about the day's topic.

BODY COACHING

DAY 15 CORTISOL

Cortisol, the main stress hormone made in your adrenal glands, has three main jobs: elevate blood sugar to feed muscles so you can run or fight, raise blood pressure, and modulate immune function. Chronically high cortisol is linked to belly fat, diabetes, high blood pressure, poor memory, depression, and insomnia.

When you're in a high-stress situation, cortisol wants sugar in your bloodstream for quick energy you can use for flight or fight. Because most of our modern-day stresses don't involve those activities, the excess sugar is stored as fat. Cortisol tells your brain you're being threatened. If this continues day after day, the brain tells your belly to start storing fat cells, and those fat cells have more cortisol receptors.[12] Scientists have found that, not only does the brain talk to the fat cells, but the fat talks back to the brain. You need to interrupt this conversation.

One of the interesting things about our spirits and cortisol is that studies have shown that praying in tongues can lower cortisol levels.[21] When we engage our personal spirits with the Holy Spirit through glossolalia —*scientist speak for praying in tongues* —our language centers of the brain are not active.[21] On brain scans the prefrontal cortex shows a reduction in activity while praying in tongues, resulting in a sense of calm and relaxation.[22]

If you'd like to try praying in tongues in addition to the body coaching, this article I (Leah) wrote has more information on how to get started. www.shelemah.com/heavens-cure-for-anxiety

Conversation Starters:

Body, I know we're in some tough situations, but these aren't the kinds of problems we need to run from. Brain, you need to adapt to a new kind of stressor; we are rarely in mortal danger. We don't need to store any more fat. In fact, the extra fat is making things seem worse than they are, so let the stress go, let the fat go, and let's all calm down.

Continue the Conversation:

Take this space to journal out any other conversations you know you need to have with your body about the day's topic.

BODY COACHING

DAY 16 STRESS

It's not hard to see how stress affects our bodies and souls. While physical stress is one aspect of the problem, most of the stress we experience really comes from emotional factors. Our bodies love to jump in on the stress party and show physical signs of emotional stress, but other than the flight-or-fight responses that keep us physically safe, our bodies don't need to become as stressed out as our souls.

In fact, if we can keep our bodies calm when undergoing emotional stress, it actually helps our minds and souls calm down and better handle the stress we are facing.

The vagus nerve plays a large role in how we respond to stress with fight, flight, or freeze. When we get stuck in a stressed response, we struggle to respond even to positive emotions and social interaction.[23] Rubbing the collarbone points shown in the tapping exercise is a great way to engage the vagus nerve and bring the body to a place of calm.

Conversation Starters:

Body, I know you feel the effects of stress that mind and soul carry. I release you from having to worry about the stress. You might feel more connected to them when you take on their burden, but you can help them get over the stress more quickly by resisting the urge to own the stress yourself. You don't have to be tense or restless.

Heart, you don't have to race. Adrenals, you don't have to produce extra cortisol. Mind and soul are well equipped to deal with stress on their end; body, you don't have to panic.

Continue the Conversation:

Take this space to journal out any other conversations you know you need to have with your body about the day's topic.

BODY COACHING

DAY 17 GAINING INSTEAD OF LOSING

If you find yourself gaining instead of losing weight, there may be one of two issues at play. Sometimes when we've done a lot to try to lose weight—dieting, restricting certain foods, cutting back our portions, exercising a ton—you actually need to eat more and put on a little weight first before it starts to come off. Not eating enough can actually stunt your metabolism, so eating more helps boost it, but you may gain before you lose.

The other thing that may be happening is that your body might be testing you. You've been saying a lot of nice things to it. Your body wants to know if all the kindness and patience is for real or if you are just trying to get what you want.

If you gain instead of lose, will you still have that kind and gentle tone, or will you revert back to the old way of bossing your body around and trying to force it to do what you want?

Conversation Starters:

Body, I'm sorry for the ways in the past that I've bossed you around and tried to force my way. I know it might not be easy to believe that this new kindness and gentleness toward you is for real, but I promise it is. I may not always talk to you or treat you perfectly, but my desire is to truly love you well and work together with you.

I understand if you need to test the waters to see if I'll revert back to old ways, but body, that hurts you just as much as it hurts me. I may slip up and revert back, but that doesn't mean that my kindness wasn't real or that we aren't making progress on working together.

Continue the Conversation:

Take this space to journal out any other conversations you know you need to have with your body about the day's topic.

BODY COACHING

DAY 18 IT'S HORMONAL

Adrenal and thyroid issues are closely linked, and the adrenals can often overcompensate for the thyroid for a while until they become burned out too. We've talked about stress and cortisol on a few different days, but today we want to speak directly to the adrenals and thyroid that are so often affected by stress and the stress hormone, cortisol.

If you know of other hormonal issues that are personally relevant, feel free to speak to those too. Thyroid and adrenal issues are really common, but other issues might need to be addressed as well.

Conversation Starters:

Body, we've been through a lot of ups and downs, and the toll those swings have taken on our adrenals and thyroid is no joke.

Adrenals, thank you for doing such a great job of managing cortisol when we need it to stay safe with fight or flight. You've gotten us through some pretty rough situations. But adrenals, it's okay to rest. You're not a victim. And we don't have to live in constant fear. If you can learn to rest in times of safety and peace, you'll be able to do an even better job when we are in dangerous situations and need you to kick in.

Thyroid, all sorts of fear is out there swirling around problems related to you—overactive, underactive—it all sounds too terrible to ever recover from. The vicious cycle of weight issues caused by thyroid issues and thyroid issues caused by weight issues further complicates matters.

Thyroid, I want to release you from all that fear. No matter what we need to do to help you be healthy, health is totally possible. Let's shake off all those fatalistic rumors we've heard about you and start living from a place of hope and patience with ourself.

Thyroid, I want you to know that I do not blame you for weight loss issues. I might have blamed you in the past, but I'm sorry for doing so. We need to address weight issues together as a whole: body—mind—spirit. It's not fair to blame you for a problem that's bigger than just one gland. No matter if you are high, low, or surgically removed, I believe we can be healthy and discover what balance is for us.

Hormones—everything from thyroid, to adrenals, to pancreas, and every endocrine gland in between—you guys have had it rough with all the work you do to keep us feeling good. Thank you all for your hard work. I want to encourage you that you were made for this work. Even if you feel like you've forgotten what you are supposed to be doing, that knowledge is deep within you in our very DNA. You've got this.

Continue the Conversation:

Take this space to journal out any other conversations you know you need to have with your body about the day's topic.

.

BODY COACHING

DAY 19 IT'S HEREDITARY

We may have told ourselves that our body type is what it is because of our genetics. Researchers in the last few years have been talking about genetic switches or dialing up or down markers that pertain to disease. Scientists in Germany found an obesity on/off switch that, when triggered, makes a lifelong epigenetically driven lean or obese state.[13] (Epigenetics refers to outside influences, such as trauma, the environment, or lifestyle changes, that affect DNA.) The fact that certain genes can be turned on or off gives us hope to make positive changes.

Aside from physical heredity, we may also have resentments towards family members that carried the unhealthy genes. As you speak to your body, also release any bitterness you've felt about your genetics. Forgive those family members; it wasn't their fault any more than it was yours. Thanks to epigenetics, we now know that we don't have to be victim to our generational biology. Just because the gene is there, doesn't mean it has to be expressed.

Conversation Starters:

Body, we've been fed some lies about genetics and hereditary weight issues. Sure, those things partially impact what we experience, but they don't have the final say. DNA, you have permission to turn off genes that are not benefiting us and wake up the dormant genes that actually help us.

Hereditary factors, you describe where I've come from but not where I am destined to go. I honor my past and my family line but do not accept hereditary health issues as normal. I forgive and release my family from being responsible for my weight.

Body, let's work together to figure out what works best for us by playing this hand that we've been dealt. No matter how bad the cards may look, I know that we can win.

Continue the Conversation:

Take this space to journal out any other conversations you know you need to have with your body about the day's topic.

BODY COACHING

DAY 20 PATIENCE

Patience, soul. If you're used to dieting and trying to boss your body around, this new approach of just talking may feel frustrating and slow. It's easy to be tempted back to old ways of restricting food groups or excessive exercising. Today is a great opportunity to remind your body and soul that slow and steady wins the race.

Conversation Starters:

Body, it's really tempting when I feel like this isn't working quickly enough to slip back into old habits. I'm sorry if I've returned to old ways of focusing too much food and trying to force you along instead of working with you gently.

Body, this new way of talking to you and being more in tune with what you're saying and needing is going to take some time to adjust to, but I'm committed to becoming more consistent with our conversations. If I revert back to old ways, you have permission to gently remind me that we need to work as a team.

Soul, I know you may feel impatient and not understand why we are being so gentle with body. You've done a lot of the talking to body for a long time now, and I need you to trust me, spirit, that I do have our best interests at heart. We need you to work with us as a team too. You do a great job of alerting me to the emotions we're feeling, but trust me to sort them out and to know how to handle them.

Continue the Conversation:

DAY 21 WHAT OTHERS HAVE SAID

Just reading today's title there are likely things that came to mind that have been said to you or about you and your body. Sadly, no one is without wounds from what others have said. It may have been your mother being well-meaning or not. You may have heard something negative from peers in school, co-workers, or so-called friends. Words might have been said to your face or been overheard as they were spoken behind your back.

No matter what was said or not said, those words hurt, and it's okay to acknowledge that hurt. Your body already knows the pain you carry, so it's a safe person to talk to about it. Ultimately, we want to forgive the people who have hurt us. Forgiveness does not mean that what they said or did was okay or that we ever have to trust them or be in relationship with them again. It just means that we are letting go of the resentments that have held our hearts captive.

As you think of specific people or groups of people that you need to forgive, the tapping exercises starting on page 27 are a great resource to help engage your body, mind, and spirit in forgiveness.

Conversation Starters:

Body, there's been a lot of things said, not said, or implied about you over the years. Even if people meant well, what they've said about you has hurt.

But body, we've been hurting long enough. Let's release the things others have said about you. Let's forgive them and choose to focus on the positive. I say that you're powerful. I say that you have amazing potential for health. I say that you're beautiful and wonderfully made. People might still say hurtful things about you from time to time, but we do not have to accept their words as truth.

Continue the Conversation:

Take this space to journal out any other conversations you know you need to have with your body about the day's topic.

BODY COACHING

DAY 22 MADE TO MOVE

Have you ever noticed how flexible toddlers are? Those yoga poses that seem impossibly out of reach for us adults are simply how little ones move around as they tumble and play. And you were once a child that could move like that too.

You might not remember it, but your body does. This belief that, as we age, we are just supposed to be less flexible and mobile isn't a biological fact. It's a cultural lie that most of us have just agreed to believe.

On top of forgetting flexibility, your body might have learned to fear movement after an injury. Tweaking that knee or rolling your ankle might have sowed a seed of doubt about the next time you try to take a step or go on that run.

We have to get over the fears that hold us back physically (while not ignoring the wise cautions) and also reject the lies that we aren't made for movement.

Conversation Starters:

Body, I know in the past we've experienced soreness and maybe even injury when we've tried to exercise and that you may be afraid of experiencing pain again.

Body, I'm sorry for any way I've ignored you when you told me to stop because you hurt. I know you might be afraid that I'll try to push you again to lose weight, or that, if we lose weight, I'll feel good and want to move you more.

But body, you were made for movement. You are magnificently designed to run, jump, stretch, twirl, climb, and do any other movement that we've ever dreamed of. I promise not to ignore you when you tell me we're doing too much too quickly, but let's start moving again in ways that feel good.

Continue the Conversation:

Take this space to journal out any other conversations you know you need to have with your body about the day's topic.

BODY COACHING

DAY 23 LIVER
AND KIDNEYS

You'll hear all sorts of things about how to do a liver or kidney cleanse to detox, but the truth is that our livers and kidneys are already perfectly designed to detoxify our bodies. Sure, you can do some things to support your liver and kidneys and help them do their jobs well, but they are the real heroes when it comes to detox - not some crazy cleanse you decided to try.

There is a lot of talk about burning fat, but have you ever wondered where in the body all that burning actually takes place? That's another thing you can thank your liver for as it plays a huge role in the metabolic process and is where fat cells get broken down and eliminated from the body through the small intestine.[14]

If excessive alcohol consumption has been an issue for you, you may also need to talk to your liver about that, giving it permission to heal and apologizing for overloading it.

Conversation Starters:

Liver and kidneys, I want to thank you guys for the hard work you do processing the junk. I'm sorry for the times I've put an unhealthy and toxic load on you. I'm also sorry for all the crazy cleanses and detoxes I've tried instead of just focusing on giving you guys what you need to do your jobs well.

Liver, I especially want to thank you for all that fat burning you do. I'm sorry that I never realized your role in that. Liver, you have permission to burn as much fat as you want, but I'll be patient as you do it at a healthy rate that our whole body can handle.

And gallbladder, I don't want to forget you either; you do such a great job managing all the bile that lets liver burn fat. I know making stones might sound like fun, but it won't be. You don't need to make anything. Your glorious purpose is to do a great job supporting liver and storing bile until it's used. No one else is as great at managing that storage as you are.

Continue the Conversation:

Take this space to journal out any other conversations you know you need to have with your body about the day's topic.

BODY COACHING

DAY 24 TRAUMATIC MEMORIES OF FOOD

You know *that* food, the one that your mom served regularly no matter how much you hated it? For me (Leah), it was green beans. Those nasty, mushy beans out of a can haunted my childhood. I know my mother meant well; she was trying to get a green vegetable into my diet. But it was years into adulthood before I even considered the fact that green beans might actually be enjoyable. I still will never eat them out of a can. But when I discovered fresh green beans roasted with a little salt, I found that the bane of my childhood meal times might not have been as totally evil as I had thought.

Other traumatic food memories may have to do with allergic responses. If that's been your experience, you'll want to talk to your body about being wise and avoiding known dangers but not fearing foods that are likely safe.

Conversation Starters:

Body, I know we have some pretty traumatic memories of foods we were forced to eat when we were younger or even foods we had an allergic response to. Let's forgive mom for feeding us food we thought was gross, even though she was just trying to help us be healthy.

Even though we thought broccoli, spinach, and green vegetables in general were not tasty when we were a kid, we've grown up now, and our taste buds might even have changed. So let's release any preconceived notions we have about healthy foods tasting bad. I'll stop saying, "Oh, I hate ____," and you can stop turning our nose up at it too.

Gag reflex, you don't need to kick in unless what we're eating really is hurting us. Let's be open to new foods and learn to enjoy the foods that give us the best nutrients.

Continue the Conversation:

Take this space to journal out any other conversations you know you need to have with your body about the day's topic.

BODY COACHING

DAY 25 SKIN

Our skin tells a lot of our stories: stretch marks from weight gained quickly, loose skin from weight lost, along with all the other scars, wrinkles, and birthmarks that tell our history. Besides being such a historian, our skin also gives indication of our current health and is often one of the first visible places we notice illness.[15]

A concern for many who have lost significant weight is having extra loose skin. Over time, our skin does tighten back up, but often not as much or as fast as we would like, so that's a great opportunity to speak to our bodies and encourage them.

Conversation Starters:

Body, one of the ways you tell me you need something is through our skin. I'm sorry if I haven't been the best are reading the signals.

Skin, I want to thank you for how hard you work to protect us, regulate our body temperature, dispose of toxins, and all the other hard work you do. I know I've stretched you beyond your limits at times, and you have been gracious to accommodate the various shapes we've taken.

Skin, I know you may be afraid of being stretched, but it's okay to tighten up. If we need you to be bigger again, you are marvelously gifted at growing. I'm going to work on appreciating every single inch of you, and you have permission to give me fewer inches to appreciate.

I also need to apologize to you, skin, for the times I've been embarrassed by you and tried to hide you, blaming you for problems that went so much further than skin deep.

Continue the Conversation:

Take this space to journal out any other conversations you know you need to have with your body about the day's topic.

BODY COACHING

DAY 26 LYMPHATIC SYSTEM

The lymphatic system circulates throughout the body, taking away toxins and waste, filtering it all through the lymph nodes, and then returning the clean fluid back to the rest of the body. The really impressive part is that the lymphatic system does all this circulating without a pump like the heart that circulates our blood stream.[16, 17]

The lymphatic system depends on our movements to circulate, so if you're spending most of your time sitting still, so is your lymph system. If you've ever seen a stagnant stream, you know how important it is to keep things flowing for health.

If moving more just isn't possible in your current situation, dry brushing is also a great way to help your lymphatic system flow better.[18]

Conversation Starters:

Body, the numerous systems you have are pretty impressive. Lymphatic system, you are an especially impressive force for health. Thank you for being such an effective garbage disposal and working so beautifully with the immune system to keep us healthy. I know you need me to move for circulation, so I'll do my best to start moving for you. But you also have permission to take a mile for every inch of movement I give you.

Continue the Conversation:

Take this space to journal out any other conversations you know you need to have with your body about the day's topic.

DAY 27 FAT

We have spent a lot of time cursing our fat. *Fat* is a bad name to call yourself or to be called, but fat also makes your brain work; supports healthy hair, nails, and skin; provides a cushion for bones and organs; offers protection, insulation, energy, and fertility; helps us absorb vitamins; produce hormones; and helps facilitate proper communication with our nerves. It's unrealistic to try to achieve two percent body-fat composition.[19]

Conversation Starters:

Body, I want to speak to our fat for a minute. Fat, you get a bad rap a lot of the time, but you play a magnificent role in: providing cushion, protection, insulation, and energy, helping us absorb vitamins, and produce hormones, and facilitating proper communication with our nerves.

Fat, please know that when we talk about wanting less of you, it's not because we don't appreciate all you do for us. We want all of us to be healthy, which includes you, but being healthy means that any extra friends you've had staying over need to go.

Continue the Conversation:

Take this space to journal out any other conversations you know you need to have with your body about the day's topic.

DAY 28 NEW NORMAL

Have you resigned yourself to the fact that weight gain as we age is just normal and that you can't do anything about it? Because if you have, that so-called *fact* is actually a lie. Biologically, there is no reason that we should have to gain weight as we age. A lot of people gain weight because of lifestyle factors, but our bodies are made to be just as healthy and trim when we age, as they were when we were younger.

Conversation Starters:

Body, we've been living under a lie, and it's time for us both to reject it. Growing older does not have to mean getting bigger. We have to pay attention to our lifestyle choices more as we age, but you are just as capable of losing weight, strengthening muscle, and being in as much overall health as you were when we were younger. Nothing is holding us back from running marathons in our 90s except our mindsets about what we can do as we age.

So body, you have permission to be as healthy as you can be for as long as we can be. Forget everything you've been told about what you can or can't do. I'm telling you that we can do anything!

Continue the Conversation:

Take this space to journal out any other conversations you know you need to have with your body about the day's topic.

DAY 29 LETTING DOWN THE DEFENSES

For some, weight has been a protection that has kept unwanted attention away, or has felt like a safe place to hide. Sexual abuse survivors commonly talk about how putting on extra weight helped them feel safe from further abuse because they didn't feel as attractive to potential abusers. Weight can also be a way that we excuse ourselves from having to participate in the parts of life that have scared or hurt us in the past.

Think back to Day 4 when we talked about what was happening when the weight gain started. Were there ways in which the weight was a welcome protection from whatever was going on?

Conversation Starters:

Body, it's time to let go of any extra weight you've been keeping to feel safe. It might have felt like protection before, but we don't need it anymore. There are better ways to protect us that won't hurt our health and ability to move and do what we want to do.

Let's reject the lie that, if we let go of the weight, we'll receive unwanted attention and will end up being hurt, that if we feel and look good, this will somehow lead to negative things. Those lies are keeping us from being healthy and are really making us miss out on a lot of fun activities.

Soul, you are so much more skilled at protecting us from hurt than some extra pounds could be. You have no need to freak out and sabotage body's attempts to lose weight. If we need protection, we have much better coping skills that won't hurt our overall health the way the weight has.

Continue the Conversation:

Take this space to journal out any other conversations you know you need to have with your body about the day's topic.

BODY COACHING

DAY 30 IT'S ONLY THE BEGINNING

Remember the *Love Letter from Your Body* on page 49 at the beginning of the book? Today is a great day to read back through that letter and remind yourself of how far you've come in building relationship with your body.

You may even want to take some time and write a love letter to your body.

While this is the end of the thirty days, you can continue conversing with your body and working together as a team—body, soul, and spirit.

Conversation Starters:

Body, today is the last day of our little experiment, but it won't be the last day that I encourage and talk gently to you. This isn't just about a thirty-day try at weight loss; it's about setting a new normal for how I interact with and speak to you. I want us to continue to be friends and work together—body, soul, and spirit.

Soul, I hope you've begun to see that you can trust me (spirit) to handle these issues. I know I'm much more gentle and patient than you would like at times, but you can rest in that patience and gentleness. I will continue being just as patient and gentle with you as I have been with body, and I'm excited to see how we grow in learning to work together as a team.

Continue the Conversation:

Take this space to journal out any other conversations you know you need to have with your body about the day's topic.

BODY COACHING

AFTER DAY 30
AND BEYOND

Woohoo! You just completed thirty days of talking to your body and learning to foster that form of communication! Our hope is, now that you've learned to talk to your body instead of just bossing it around, that this new gentler approach will become normal for you; and that going back to the old ways of doing things just won't appeal to you anymore. We hope that you'll continue to grow in all areas of life with spirit taking the lead over soul and body.

You have some options from here on out:

- You can repeat the thirty days as often as you want
- You can keep talking to your body on your own now that you know how this works
- You can page back through to find the areas that really resonated with you as what you need to work on with your body
- You can begin making healthy lifestyle shifts as you talk to your body

We have covered some broad ground, and now you can specialize. I might also suggest following or subscribing to some smart and sane health publications and use the information as inspiration for talking to your body. For basic information on how the different body systems and organs work, check out PubMed Health online.[20]

Healthy & Whole

If you're ready to begin making some lifestyle shifts toward health in addition to talking to yourself, Leah's book, *Healthy & Whole: 60 Days to Complete Wellness*, will help you build sustainable healthy habits in body—mind—spirit.

No matter where you are in your health journey, Leah's book meets you where you're at and adds healthy practices at a pace you can keep up with. You can even do *Healthy & Whole* while going back through the *Body Coaching* conversations.

RECOMMENDED RESOURCES

Books:

Healthy & Whole: 60 Days to Complete Wellness by Leah Lesesne

Think and Eat Yourself Smart by Dr. Caroline Leaf

Wrecked: Why Your Quest For Health And Weight Loss Has Failed...And What You Can Do About It by Dr. Steven Prentice

Forever Fat Loss by Ari Whitten

Websites:

Eat Like a Normal Person
www.eatlikeanormalperson.com

Igniting Hope Ministries
www.ignitinghope.com

Captive Thought Therapy
www.captivethoughttherapy.com

BODY COACHING

REFERENCES

1. Philip Werdell, "Physical Craving and Food Addiction: A Scientific Review," *Food Addiction Institute,* accessed March 2, 2018, https://foodaddictioninstitute.org/scientific-research/physical-craving-and-food-addiction-a-scientific-review/.

2. Caroline Leaf, M. D., "Gut-Brain Connection," *Dr. Leaf's Blog,* November 23, 2016, accessed March 2, 2018, https://drleaf.com/blog/gut-brain-connection/.

3. Janet Epping, "Leptin Resistance May Block The 'Full' Message And Lead To Obesity," *Medical News Today,* March 3, 2011, accessed March 2, 2018, https://www.medicalnewstoday.com/articles/217958.php.

4. Megan Stevens, "5 Ways To Heal Your Gut That You Probably Haven't Tried," *Traditional Cooking School,* June 25, 2017, accessed March 2, 2018, https://traditionalcookingschool.com/health-and-nutrition/5-ways-heal-gut-probably-havent-tried/.

5. Michael F. Picco, M.D., "Digestion: How long does it take?" *Mayo Clinic,* January 18, 2018, accessed March 2, 2018, https://www.mayoclinic.org/digestive-system/expert-answers/faq-20058340.

6. Ritamarie Loscalzo, "Hypoglycemia and the Myth of Eating Frequent Small Meals," *Dr. Ritamarie*, accessed March 2, 2018, http://drritamarie.com/blog/hypoglycemia-and-the-myth-of-eating-frequent-small-meals/.

7. John Douillard, "Sleep Interrupted? The Blood Sugar and Sleep Connection," *LifeSpa*, January 19, 2012, accessed March 2, 2018, https://lifespa.com/sleep-interrupted-the-blood-sugar-and-sleep-connection/.

8. Janet Epping, "Leptin Resistance May Block The 'Full' Message And Lead To Obesity,"

9. Barry M. Popkin, Kristen E. D'Anci, and Irwin H. Rosenberg, "Water, Hydration and Health," *US National Library of Medicine National Institutes of Health*, August 1, 2011, accessed March 2, 2018, https://www.ncbi.nlm.nih.gov/pmc/articles/PMC2908954/.

10. Marge Dwyer, "Study finds inadequate hydration among U.S. children," *Harvard T.H. Chan School of Public Health*, accessed March 2, 2018, https://www.hsph.harvard.edu/news/press-releases/study-finds-inadequate-hydration-among-u-s-children/.

11. Staff, "How do the kidneys work?" *US National Library of Medicine National Institutes of Health*, January 7, 2015, accessed March 2, 2018,

https://www.ncbi.nlm.nih.gov/pubmedhealth/PM
H0072569/.

12. University of Florida, "Body fat can send signals to brain, affecting stress response," July 23, 2015, accessed March 2, 2018, https://www.sciencedaily.com/releases/2015/07/150723111359.htm?trendmd-shared=0.

13. Karen Dalgaard, et al., "Trim28 Haploinsufficiency Triggers Bi-stable Epigenetic Obesity," *Cell*, January 28, 2016, accessed March 2, 2018, Vol. 164, Issue 3, 353–364, http://www.cell.com/cell/fulltext/S0092-8674(15)01689-X.

14. Staff, "How does the liver work?" *US National Library of Medicine National Institutes of Health*, August 22, 2016, accessed March 2, 2018, https://www.ncbi.nlm.nih.gov/pubmedhealth/PM H0072577/.

15. Staff, "How does skin work?" *US National Library of Medicine National Institutes of Health*, July 28, 2016, accessed March 2, 2018, https://www.ncbi.nlm.nih.gov/pubmedhealth/PM H0072439/.

16. Staff, "Lymphatic System," *US National Library of Medicine National Institutes of Health*, accessed March 2, 2018, https://www.ncbi.nlm.nih.gov/pubmedhealth/PM HT0024459/.

17. Inho Choi, et al., "The New Era of the Lymphatic
     System: No Longer Secondary to the Blood
     Vascular System," *US National Library of
     Medicine National Institutes of Health*, April
     2012, accessed March 2, 2018, Vol. 2, Issue 4,
     https://www.ncbi.nlm.nih.gov/pmc/articles/PMC
     3312397/.

18. Staff, "Dry Brushing for Skin, Circulatory, and
     Lymphatic Health," *Shelemah body-mind-spirit*,
     August 8, 2017, Accessed March 2, 2018,
     http://shelemah.com/dry-brushing-for-skin-
     circulatory-and-lymphatic-health/.

19. Staff, "Body Fat – How Does It Affect Health?"
     HealthStatus, accessed March 2, 2018,
     https://www.healthstatus.com/health_blog/body-
     fat-calculator-2/body-fat-how-does-it-affect-
     health/.

20. "Browse For Consumers - National Library of
     Medicine - PubMed Health." National Center for
     Biotechnology Information. Accessed March 02,
     2018.
     https://www.ncbi.nlm.nih.gov/pubmedhealth/s/f
     or_consumers_medrev/a/.

21. Lynn, Christopher Dana, et al. "Salivary Alpha-
     Amylase and Cortisol among Pentecostals on a
     Worship and Nonworship Day." *American
     Journal of Human Biology*, vol. 22, no. 6, 2010,
     pp. 819–822., doi:10.1002/ajhb.21088.

22. Francis, Leslie J. "Personality and Glossolalia: A Study Among Male Evangelical Clergy." *Pastoral Psychology*, vol. 51, no. 5, 2003, pp. 391–396., doi:10.1023/a:1023618715407.

23. Rosenberg, Stanley. *Accessing the Healing Power of the Vagus Nerve: Self-Help Exercises for Anxiety, Depression, Trauma, and Autism.* North Atlantic Books, 2016.

BODY COACHING

OTHER BOOKS BY THE AUTHORS

Healthy & Whole: 60 Days to Complete Wellness by Leah Lesesne

Healing in the Hebrew Months Book One: A Biblical Understanding of Each Season's Emotional Healing by Leah Lesesne

Healing in the Hebrew Months Book Two: Prophetic Strategies Hidden in the Tribes, Constellations, Gates, and Gems by Seneca Schurbon

Broken to Whole: Inner Healing for the Fragmented Soul by Seneca Schurbon, et al.

Accessing Your Spiritual Inheritance by Seneca Schurbon, Del Hungerford, and Alice Briggs

Flower Power: Essences that Heal by Seneca Schurbon

OTHER BOOKS BY THE AUTHORS

ABOUT THE AUTHORS

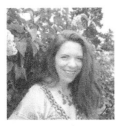

Seneca Schurbon

Seneca is the founder and chief experimenter at Freedom Flowers. She boldly pushes the limits, weaving the natural and the spiritual together, and is passionate about helping people find their healing breakthroughs.

FB: www.facebook.com/freedomfloweressence
Instagram: @FreedomFlowerEssence
Website: www.Freedom-Flowers.com

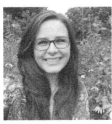

Leah Lesesne

Leah is an inner healing practitioner with a masters in professional counseling. She is the creator of Captive Thought Therapy and loves bringing together her counseling and inner healing skill sets to help you be as healthy, whole, and close to Jesus as possible.

FB: www.facebook.com/shelemahwellness
Instagram: @ShelemahWellness
Website: www.Shelemah.com

GET THE BODY COACHING WEIGHT LOSS PROGRAM FROM FREEDOM FLOWERS

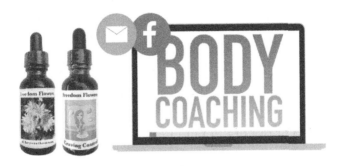

http://bit.ly/BCKit

Program Kit Includes:

- Email reminders of the daily conversation starters
- Membership in an exclusive Facebook group and the support of others doing Body Coaching
- A bottle of Chrysanthemum flower essence, and
- A bottle of Craving Control flower essence blend

Made in the USA
Monee, IL
29 December 2020